purify

To my va va voom women - bodi.

May this provide moe inspiration on your dedicated path!

With love and support

fellow va va voom chica

♡ Jaulie

January 2006

purify

101 ways to detox

Elisabeth Wilson

MQP

Dedication
For my dear friend Anna Pank. With whom I've detoxed many times, but re-toxed more often.

Published by MQ Publications Limited
12 The Ivories, 6-8 Northampton Street
London N1 2HY
Tel: 020 7359 2244
Fax: 020 7359 1616
email: mail@mqpublications.com
website: www.mqpublications.com

Series Editor: Karen Ball, MQ Publications
Editorial Director: Ljiljana Baird, MQ Publications
Senior Designer: Victoria Bevan, MQ Publications
Design concept by Balley Design Associates
Photography by Stuart Boreham

ISBN 1-84072-588-5

Printed in France by *Partenaires-Livres*® (JL)

1 3 5 7 9 0 8 6 4 2

Caution
Aromatherapy oils should not be placed directly on the skin and should always be diluted. Women who are pregnant or hoping to become pregnant, or people suffering from any medical condition, have circulatory disease or diabetes should seek medical advice before undertaking any of the recommendations in this book.

This book is intended as an informational guide only and is not to be used as a substitute for professional medical care or treatment. Neither the author nor the publisher can be held responsible for any damage, injury, or otherwise resulting from the use of the information in this book.

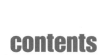

contents

Introduction

Detoxify. What does it mean to you? Self-sacrifice? Misery? A month of eating brown rice and mung beans?

There is a place for that sort of detoxing but this book isn't it. Here we recognize that in the real world time is precious. What you need are proven methods of purifying that make the detoxing process easy, and above all, pleasurable— because if you don't really want to do it, you probably won't.

Experts argue about just how toxic our environment is and whether detoxing is indeed necessary. Our view is that whether you live in an inner city or breathe the purer air of the country, detoxing is simply self-nurturing by another name and we can all benefit from taking time to look after our bodies to help them function optimally. The rewards are clearer skin, sparkling eyes, and looking and feeling lighter and brighter. You'll have more energy immediately, and the long-term gain from eating good food is a more efficient immune system which means less illness.

All this for minimal input. If you have only ten minutes, each of the 101 suggestions in this book is in itself a mini-miracle—a mind or body detoxifying treatment that will leave you feeling both energized and relaxed almost instantly. To ensure that you achieve the most in the quickest time, the 101 ideas are grouped into seven different detoxing "days"—one to suit every need or mood. With a weekend or a week to spare, you can pick and mix several "days" to create your customized detoxifying program.

Each section also has its own "Instant detox" tips, so that if you only have time to look at one tip a day, this is the one that will immediately help you feel better about your health and your life.

You won't find any obscure ingredients, boring diet regimes, or strict rules. Rigid adherence to the suggestions here isn't necessary. Don't fancy a particular suggestion? Fine, skip it. Or customize so that it's still healthy but more your kind of thing.

You don't have to spend a fortune on fancy spa holidays or expensive products to get detox benefits. All you need is a warm bathroom and the desire to indulge.

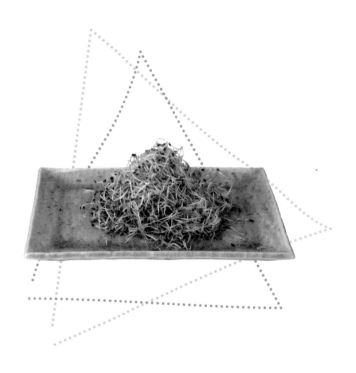

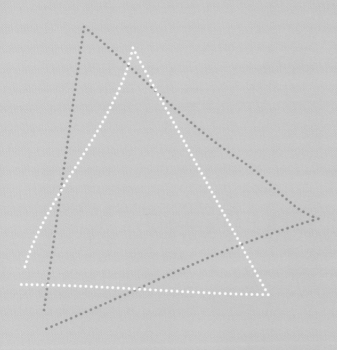

The essentials

Every day of your detox—better still, every
day of your life—make time for these
health-promoting habits.

1 Body brushing

Warning! After a few days body brushing becomes totally addictive: showering without body brushing feels akin to brushing your teeth without the toothpaste.

Body brushing—or dry skin brushing—is a more intense form of exfoliation than if you use an exfoliating gel or cream with water. Brushing your body clears away debris from the biggest organ of detoxification—your skin. Before your daily shower or bath, use a soft, natural-bristle brush on your skin, working from the soles of your feet upward and inward toward your heart (skipping your face and chest). This will exfoliate any dead skin cells, improve circulation, and encourage the lymph flow that drains away waste.

2 Hot lemon water

First thing in the morning, drink a glass of hot water into which you've squeezed the juice of half a lemon.

Not only will this wake you up, but you're also doing your body a favor! Everything you eat and drink is processed by the liver which is the most important detoxifying organ. The liver works through the night to cleanse your body, so drinking hot lemon water first thing in the morning helps your body complete the job of detoxification. (Lemon juice is a traditional agent for cleansing.) Go somewhere quiet and peaceful to drink your lemon water, back to bed or the garden. This is your oasis of calm before the day starts.

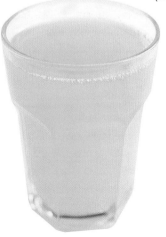

3 Space

To keep sane you need "down-time" when your mind can switch off and your body simply flop. There is plenty of time unaccounted for in our programs; it's there for you to relax, kick back, watch favorite movies, read novels, write in your journal, stare into the fire, and dream. "Space" is not watching TV or reading the newspaper or listening to the radio. These drain rather than restore energy. On the other hand, "space" is the perfect place for lying on the couch and really listening to your CD collection.

4 Instant detox [1]

Detox your diary. People can be toxic, too. Scan your appointments for the next month and try to cancel anyone who doesn't make you feel good about life or good about yourself. Watch your energy soar over the coming weeks. Think carefully about those you choose to spend your time with in the future.

5 Stretch

Just think how well your body serves you, so much of the time, with absolutely no acknowledgment for all its hard work. Exercise is your body's idea of double chocolate sundae. Indulge it. Once a day try a few stretches or a gentle walk. A little exercise will help put you in touch with what your body is trying to tell you. Listening to your body is a good habit to get into.

6 Drink water

We need fluid to function. Good, old-fashioned water is best because unlike just about any other fluid you can think of from orange juice to ouzo, it doesn't have any potential adverse effects. Don't wait until you feel thirsty as even mild dehydration can cause lethargy. Drinking four to eight glasses of water a day will give you energy. Ideally, choose distilled, filtered, or a good-quality mineral water.

Don't forget that many fruit and vegetables have a high water content—which is even more of a reason to turn to fresh food.

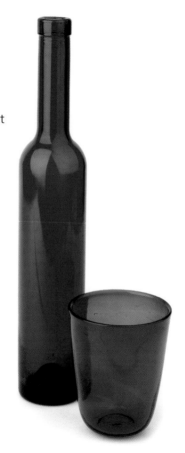

7 Early nights

Sleep allows a daily "spring clean" of your major organs, which is why it is so vital to good health. Hormones "wash out" your system, especially in the first few hours of sleep. Make a point of being in bed by 9.30P.M. when you are detoxing (even if you can't fall asleep straightaway).

You should also listen to your body during the day. It is no coincidence that you often find yourself feeling sleepy in the afternoons—the body naturally wants to take a nap at that time of day. A short nap can make all the difference to your energy resources, so don't feel guilty about getting a bit of extra shut-eye during the day.

The constants

You do have to give up some things if you want to feel better. This is often where people first falter with a detox regime, but stay positive. Just remember—you usually have to work for anything worth having in life, and detoxing is a great way of realizing that you're not as hooked on "baddies" as you thought you were. Try the following to help you resist any sudden cravings:

Plan ahead. Try to stock up on all the organic, natural foods you will want to eat as part of your detox.

Put temptation out of the way. All those high processed foods you normally snack on should be hidden far from sight.

Forgive yourself. Your first detox will be a learning process. If you weaken at any point, don't give up on the whole program. Just put it down to experience and move on.

8 Remember man-made is bad

Give your body a break. As a rule, any man-made food is harder work for your body to process than food in its natural state. Avoiding, even just for a short time, all processed food including bread, pasta, ready meals, cakes, cookies, candy, and anything with artificial additives, does wonders for energy levels. Work on developing a taste for the sort of foods recommended here, brimming as they are with antioxidant vitamins and minerals to hoover up the toxic by-products that cause disease.

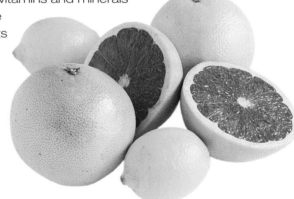

9 Food is a drug

Chinese doctors treat caffeine with great respect and use it in small medicinal doses as a tonic—they're horrified by our Western habit of guzzling it on every occasion. Certain foodstuffs have a powerful effect on our body and can induce cravings. While you detox, out of bounds are caffeine (including tea, coffee, and chocolate), alcohol, and sugar. We'll include nicotine here as well because it has a similar effect. See detoxing as an opportunity for discovering how much calmer you are without those food-induced swings in blood sugar levels that ultimately sap your energy.

10 Protein gives energy

Traditional detoxes exclude protein but a small amount of protein foods (white meat and oily fish) are included in some of our programs because they are a good, long-lasting source of energy and stop you feeling hungry. Since the main idea is to make you feel fabulous, they have their place in our detox. If you are vegetarian, use beans, legumes, nuts, or tofu as a substitute in recipes, or simply skip the protein as the meals are packed with nutrients without it.

11 Don't get too good, too quickly

You will have to eschew alcohol, soft drinks, caffeinated tea, and coffee to get the best results, but if you normally drink a lot of these (more than three cups a day), please reduce the amount you drink gradually or you risk feeling awful rather than great. At least three days before you start, begin to replace "bad" drinks with herbal equivalents. Rooibosch (Redbush tea) is a strong-tasting, caffeine-free tea packed with cancer-beating antioxidants, and it has more "bite" than normal herbal teas so you don't feel you're making such a sacrifice. The rule of gradual elimination applies to cigarettes, too.

12 Instant detox [2]

What's the simplest way to feel on top of things and in control? Dejunk your life. The Eastern "science of placement" known as feng shui teaches that physical clutter saps energy as surely as too much high living. As an experiment, throw away, give away, or donate to charity something you no longer use or need today and every day for the next seven days. In addition, use any spare five minutes to organize a drawer, declutter your handbag or reorganize your wallet by throwing out all those old receipts. Little steps like this will lift your energy significantly over the next few days.

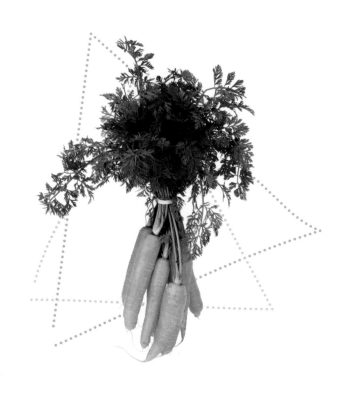

Glow

Choose this program when you feel tired and look drawn . . . when you want to smooth away visible signs of stress and restore radiance to your looks . . . when you're desperate for a vacation.

It erases signs of strain with deep-cleansing treatments based on exfoliation. This means sloughing away dead skin cells, promoting growth of new ones and thus improving circulation—which in turn encourages oxygen flow to the skin. You will also be eating foods that provide essential support for cellular regeneration.

By tomorrow you will feel shiny and new. Sparkling—inside and out.

13 "Right here, right now" meditation

Get outside and simply breathe. When your mind starts whirring with thoughts, gently bring its attention back to what you can see, hear, and feel. Note the breeze on your face, the song of the birds. Stop and examine in detail anything beautiful that catches your attention. Welcome to the state of "mindfulness" —being here is a form of meditation. With practice you will be able to slip into mindfulness whenever life's stresses threaten to overwhelm you.

14 Breakfast: pink restorer

This excellent juice is great for exhaustion as it's packed with antioxidants but is still very soothing. Blend 1 punnet of raspberries (or equivalent berries defrosted) with the flesh of 2 peaches and 1 apple. Sip slowly. (It is a thick juice, so dilute with water or orange juice if you prefer.)

15 Soothing honey hair mask

This is a rich moisturizing treatment for hair. Honey is healing and nourishing while rosemary and lavender essential oils are known for their scalp-soothing properties. You will need 2 tbsp clear honey, 1 tbsp almond or other base oil, 1 egg yolk, 3 drops rosemary essential oil, 3 drops lavender essential oil, and a plastic haircap. Combine the ingredients. Bend forward and give your hair a good brush to "loosen" the scalp. Then wet hair, towel dry, and apply the mask to scalp and hair. Put on the cap and wrap your head in a towel. Wait at least 30 minutes before shampooing off in cool water (you could try the energy sweep on the next page while you are waiting for the mask to work).

16 Energy sweep

This is a Chinese exercise to restore energy levels at any time during the day. Go as fast or as slow as you like. It works well if you start slowly, then with subsequent repetitions build up speed. Breathe evenly but normally throughout. Stand with your feet apart, knees slightly bent and arms held with elbows out and palms facing into the chest. Stretch your arms out to the side so the palms face forward, then take your hands back to cradle the back of your head. Sweep your hands down your neck, over your shoulders, and down your chest, and rest the palms on your ribcage. Take your hands to the back so each is over a kidney above the buttocks. Now sweep the palms over your hips and down the outside of your legs, over your feet, and up the inside of your legs, finally bringing both hands to rest one on top of each other just under your navel. Repeat ten times.

17 Choose ginseng to restore balance

Ginseng is what is known as an adaptogenic herb: it acts as needed to help the body cope with physical or mental stress, probably by affecting the hormones that control our stress responses. Athletes take it a few days before a big event to help bring them to peak performance. Studies have shown that students taking 400mg a day before exams remembered more information. Try taking a supplement supplying 500–1000mg of ginseng today and for the next three weeks before food. It should be taken only in short bursts of no longer than three weeks or the body adapts to it.

18 Seaweed wrap and restorative sea meditation

Rest is an intrinsic part of this treatment so find a place in your home where you can be completely undisturbed for at least an hour. Lay two heavy blankets on a bed or couch. Cover with an old, clean sheet. Play a CD of wave sounds or burn an oceanic scented candle to heighten the effect. Next, in the bathroom, apply a seaweed-based body mask (from a health store) to boost circulation and improve skin tone. (Alternatively, you can use any mask designed for this purpose.) Leave it to dry for a minute or so. Then, making sure that any candles are burning safely, snuggle down, wrapping yourself in first the sheet and then the blankets, the tighter the better (enlist help if necessary). Make sure your feet are tightly wrapped and put a towel around your head. Only your face should be uncovered. Relax for at least 30 minutes. Drink plenty of water before and after because salt and seaweed treatments are dehydrating.

19 Salt scrub

A salt scrub is an age-old
way of sloughing off old
skin cells so that new
skin can emerge. You
will need two grades
of salt: fine table salt
for your face (take
care near the eye
area) and rock salt for
your body. In one bowl
combine into a paste 2 tbsp
fine salt with half a tbsp olive oil. In
another bowl, combine into a smooth paste a handful of natural
rock salt, 1 tbsp olive oil, and a drop or two of lavender essential
oil if you wish. First body brush (see Tip 1). Then take an almost-
hot shower to relax your muscles. Turn off the shower, then
gently rub the fine-salt paste over your face and the rock-salt
paste over your body. You may need some extra rock salt,
so have it to hand. Rinse off with warm water and towel
yourself dry briskly.

20 Lunch: multivitamin soup

Vegetables and pulses are packed with the kind of fiber that lowers cholesterol and helps the body eliminate waste products efficiently. They also supply a great big blast of antioxidant vitamins that will help your body repair the ravages wrought by a frantic lifestyle. Put 4½oz split red lentils, half a leek, 1 carrot, 1 celery stick, and 1 garlic clove (all chopped) in 1 U.S. pint (500ml) vegetable stock. Bring to the boil then simmer for 20–30 minutes or until the ingredients are mushy. Remove from the heat and blend. Reheat gently and serve with a scattering of herbs such as parsley and a grind of black pepper.

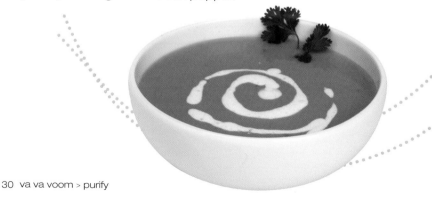

21 Mellow stone meditation

This treatment locates acupressure points on your face and helps release muscle tension. You will need five small stones, smooth on one side so that they will balance on your face. Place them in a bowl of boiling water for ten minutes to cleanse and warm them. Remove them with a spoon and pat them dry. Now work quickly. Lie down in a comfortable, quiet room and place one stone centrally in the middle of your forehead below the browline, another between your eyebrows on the "third eye," one more in the dent below your lower lip on your chin, and two on either side of your nose by the nostrils. Breathing evenly, take your concentration from one stone to the other and imagine the warmth that is penetrating your skin from the stones activating skin renewal. Rest like this until the stones have cooled.

22 The centering facial

This is a way of bringing a sense of ritual to the most mundane task and it helps shift you into a contemplative, quiet "place" before bed. You will need a creamy facial cleanser, cottonwool, your favorite night moisturizer, and a mirror. Apply the cleanser liberally, then sweep it away with cottonwool. Look at your reflection steadily in the mirror while mentally running through the day, revisiting the highs and lows. Splash your face with warm water. Then consciously let the worries of the day go, draining away with the water. Next apply moisturizer and, using your middle fingers, massage it into your skin, all the while holding your gaze in the mirror. As you do so, remember the good points of the day and feel the warmth of any successes. Finish by cupping your hands over your face and inhaling any fragrance deeply. As you exhale, let this day go.

23 Dinner: uplifting salad

This salad provides a combination of omega-3 oils (from the salmon) and omega-6 oils (from the walnuts), which is a winning combination for your heart but also does wonders for your mood and your skin. Chop or crush a handful of walnuts. Grill a tuna steak in a little rapeseed oil. Make a salad dressing from walnut oil, vinegar, and black pepper. Drizzle the dressing over a large bowl of mixed green salad leaves and toss, along with the crushed walnuts. Place the tuna on top of the leaves and eat straight away.

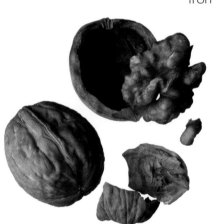

24 Instant detox [3]

Try an overnight mini-fast.
Don't eat anything and
sip only water after 6pm
in the evening. Next
morning have just
a fruit or vegetable
juice for breakfast
(see Chapter 5,
Purify for ideas),
then only water
until a light lunch
of, say, a salad or
soup. You'll have
gone around 14 hours
without loading up your
stomach and should feel
better for it. This is good when
you've eaten too much rich food.

Recharge

Choose this program when just getting out of bed is an effort . . . when you have too much to think about, too much to do . . . when you've lost your zest for life.

The ideal food combination when you're exhausted is the one suggested here: protein for long-lasting energy release and plenty of the sort of carbohydrates that won't cause mad swings in your blood sugar and lead to energy slumps.

By tomorrow you will feel refreshed, revitalized, and raring to go.

25 Breakfast: saintly muesli (requires pre-preparation)

You will need 1 cup organic oatmeal, 2 tbsp sultanas, 4 tbsp apple juice, 1 apple, and 1 tbsp chopped almonds. Soak the oatmeal and sultanas in the juice overnight. Next morning grate in the apple, sprinkle in the almonds, and serve with a dollop of live natural yogurt.

26 Clear the clutter

Even if you think you thrive on chaos, a cluttered, disorganized space weighs on your mind and affects your ability to get things done. Everything takes longer if your living space isn't streamlined. Take an hour this morning to straighten your home, throwing out whatever is no longer needed. (If this would take much longer than an hour, make sure the rooms to be used today are tidy. Then do yourself a favor and set aside a weekend in your diary to deal with the rest.)

27 Space clearing

Bring fresh vibrations into your home and you'll feel that the atmosphere is more supportive of your well-being. Here is a tried and tested method of literally clearing the air. Throw open the windows and walk around your (tidy!) home ringing a little handbell gently or vigorously as the mood takes you. (Your intuition will tell you what's needed.) Clap your hands if you don't have a bell. Be especially careful to ring or clap under furniture and in corners. You may well feel self-conscious at first, but remember that every major world religion uses sound—usually bells—to mark out a space as sacred. When you have finished, light a fragrant candle, aromatherapy burner, or incense stick to heighten the sense that something important is about to happen. Which indeed it is.

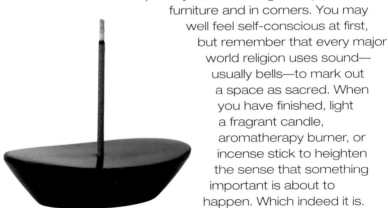

28 Flash shower

Challenging but marvelous, hydrotherapy is the name for treatments that use alternate shots of hot and cold water to wake up your circulatory system. This boosts your immune system, encourages blood and oxygen flow—and wakes you up like nothing else. First body brush (see Tip 1). Next take a warm shower. After a few minutes, switch to cold water. Do this gradually or instantly (some people find the latter easier) but the water has to be cold. Let it cascade over you for ten seconds. No cheating! You'll feel like yowling, but try your hardest to relax. Switch back to warm for a minute. Then back to cold for ten seconds. Repeat again so that you sluice with cold water a total of three times. Finish with a warm shower and then jump out and towel yourself dry vigorously. Yes, it's tough— but a small price to pay for feeling this good.

29 Energizing drench

A wonderful end to every shower but
especially the one opposite, the
drench will set you up for the rest of
the day. You will need a mister
(available from chemists or
at a pinch use those
sold to gardeners for
misting plants), olive
oil, and an energizing
aromatherapy essential oil
(try rosemary, grapefruit, or
bergamot). Add 1 teaspoon olive oil to
7 tbsp water plus a few drops of your chosen
essential oil. Mix well then mist generously over your body.
Allow to dry naturally on your bare skin, inhaling the
invigorating fragrance.

30 Instant detox [4]

Some electrical equipment such as photocopiers and printers give off volatile organic compounds (VOCs) that can lead to symptoms such as fatigue, headaches, and lack of concentration. However, NASA scientists have discovered that you can detox your office space by adding greenery, notably spider plants and aloe vera, which neutralize the effects of VOCs. Peace lilies are also especially good at absorbing and recycling stale air.

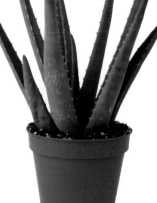

31 Power walk

Walking briskly, forcefully, powerfully is a totally different experience from ambling along. It counts as aerobic exercise and speeds up the detoxing process by encouraging body organs to work more efficiently. Also—trust us—you'll feel more energetic afterward. Find somewhere leafy. Start by doing a few simple calf stretches. Now off you go. Don't overstride—take normal steps but go faster than normal. Bend your elbows and swing your arms to increase the blood flow. Allow your stride to roll from your heel through to your toe. Be conscious of the breath flowing in and out of your body as you inhale deeply through your nose. Keep going for at least 20 minutes. By the end you should be pink and panting but not uncomfortably so.

32 Egg nourishing mask

This is an instant face lift, tightening and lifting, so skin feels nicely taut. You will need 1 egg and 1 tbsp sunflower (or olive) oil. Blend them together well, then massage into your skin. Leave for 20 minutes. Rinse off with warm water. Your skin will be baby soft.

33 Lunch: tonic salad

This supplies essential omega-3 oils (good for lifting mood and just about everything else) and vitamin E from the nuts to give you energy and fight off the physical side effects of exhaustion. Crush or chop a handful of hazelnuts. Make a large mixed leaf salad and a dressing of balsamic vinegar and olive oil. Toss these together gently with the hazelnuts. Grill a salmon steak or fillet, place it on the salad, and serve immediately with a wedge of lime.

34 "Ain't life grand?" mood booster

Feel in a rut? This mental exercise frees you up fast and shows you that a more focused, happier life can be yours, starting tomorrow. The secret is to think laterally.

Brew a cup of peppermint tea (good for clearing your mind). Take it, and a notebook and pen, to a quiet spot. Close your eyes and imagine what a perfect day in your life would look like. Reality and "yes, buts" have no place here. A tropical beach? A day in bed with an adoring lover? A book tour promoting your bestselling novel? Write it all out in detail. Now examine what you've written, looking at what your desires say about how you would like to feel. The above examples could translate into feeling relaxed in the sun with nothing to worry about, feeling loved, or feeling successful. Then resolve to take steps to get away for a break; cherish yourself (if there's no one else about to do it); or boost your self-esteem. Those feelings (if not the actual dreams just yet) are all potentially achievable by tomorrow.

35 Take the energy pill

Coenzyme Q10 is a natural substance found in the body that speeds up metabolic processes, notably those affecting energy levels and body repair. It also has strong antioxidant properties, working with vitamins C and E to reduce damage produced by pollution, smoking, and passive smoking. You can get it from food—notably mackerel, sardines, and soya beans—but to increase intake enough to see marked improvement you should take a supplement. Starting today, aim for 50mg twice a day; you will see energy levels and immunity improve in about a month.

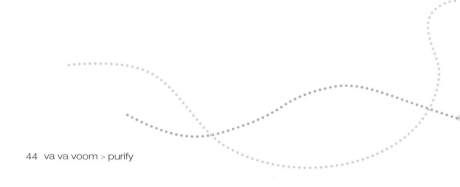

36 Dinner: jumping bean soup

Beans and pulses contain the sort of fiber that helps the body remove toxins and they are also a super source of energy. The vegetables make this a powerful antioxidant soup, too.

Drain a medium can of flageolet (or cannellini) beans and put them in a saucepan with 1 U.S. pint (500ml) vegetable stock. Bring to the boil and let simmer in a covered pan while you gently fry in a large frying pan a little olive oil, half an onion, and 1 garlic clove. Add half a cabbage (chopped) when the onion is soft and fry for a few more minutes. Add the beans with their cooking water. Cook for another 15 minutes. Season and add fresh chopped parsley. Liquidize if preferred.

37 Epsom bath

This is one of the most purifying and powerful detoxing methods available to you. It also helps you sleep. You will need 4½lb (2kg) Epsom salts (or Dead Sea salts) available from chemists and health food stores, a glass of still water, and candles. Run a warm bath, pour in the salts, and make sure that they have all dissolved—you may have to stir. The salts promote sweating so you must take care not to become dehydrated. Relax in the bath, sipping water at intervals, then use a loofah or sisal glove to massage your skin slowly from the tip of your toes up to your neck. Stay in the bath for at least 20 minutes. Emerge and wrap yourself in warm towels. Take care to wear a plaster over any small scratches or the salt will sting. Don't take an Epsom bath if you have diabetes or a heart condition.

Rejuvenate

Choose this program when you want
to put back the clock . . . when you
deserve a treat . . . when you want
to luxuriate.

It will smooth, soothe, and nourish your
body back to peak condition. The meals
are packed full of the nutrients—vitamins
A, C, and E—that keep you looking young
and feeling healthy.

By tomorrow you won't just feel
good, you'll look good.

38 Breakfast: warming fruit compote (requires pre-preparation)

This is rich in antioxidants in general, and vitamin E in particular, which makes it terrific for skin. Combine 4½oz (125g) dried fruit (such as apricots, figs, and prunes) with ¼ U.S. pint (150ml) orange juice and leave to soak overnight. Simmer the fruits gently for ten minutes and serve with natural yogurt and finely grated almonds.

39 Double-cream exfoliation

Gentle rubbing (exfoliation) makes the skin look younger and more refined. Women have been using oatmeal to do this for thousands of years, and this treatment leaves skin baby-soft thanks to the double cream. Combine 1 tbsp fine oatmeal and 1 tbsp double cream. Rub the mixture lightly into your clean face and neck using the pads of your fingers, avoiding the eyes. Rinse off with warm water, and sweep off any last remnants with cotton wool.

40 Fragrant deep-conditioning oil infusion for hair

Sandalwood is deeply moisturizing, sensual, warming, and relaxing. You will need 1tbsp sunflower or almond oil mixed with 3 drops sandalwood essential oil, a plastic shower cap, and an old towel. Brush your hair, thoroughly "loosening" the scalp. Strip to the waist or wear an old T-shirt (the oil will drip). Massage the oil infusion with your fingertips slowly into your scalp and down the length of your hair, making small, circular movements with your fingertips. If your scalp is oily, do only the hair. Put on the plastic cap for 30 minutes (or if you prefer until you've completed the two treatments below). Then shampoo the oil away—it may take two applications of shampoo. Let hair dry naturally.

41 Strawberry-smoothie body mask

Fruits, especially strawberries, are loaded with naturally occurring alpha-hydroxy acids (AHAs) that exfoliate the skin and soften it. You will need 1 punnet of strawberries, 1 lemon to squeeze, 2 peaches (skin intact), 1 mango, 1 banana, a large bowl, and at least three old towels. Make sure that your bathroom is warm. Pulp all the fruits in the bowl until you have a gooey paste. Step onto an old towel or into the bath or shower and smear the pulp over your body and face. Wrap yourself in the other two towels and wait at least five minutes for the fruit to do its work. Shower off with warm water and dry yourself well. (Wash towels immediately.)

42 Yogurt body dip

When skin is completely dry after the smoothie body mask, cleanse and nourish it with this treatment. You will need 1 large pot of natural yogurt, a small or medium paintbrush, and an old towel. Paint the yogurt all over your body with the paintbrush. Use fingers to apply it to your face. The sensation of the yogurt on your skin will be cool and relaxing. Wait five minutes then shower off in warm water. If you're a little cold after the last two treatments, warm up with a luxuriating bath scented with a few drops of your favorite essential oil and slip back into bed until lunchtime.

43 Lunch: skin-saving fish dish

Salmon increases the skin's water-holding capacity, so it plumps it up and promotes smooth, soft skin. Avocado is a superb source of vitamin E, renowned for its skin-boosting ability. Gently fry a salmon fillet in olive oil. While it is cooking, mash 1 avocado and mix it with 3 tsps live natural yogurt and a grind of black pepper. When the salmon is ready, serve it with a dollop or large spoonful of avocado over it, garnished with chopped spring onions, and a large green salad.

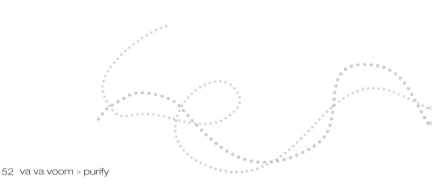

44 Avocado face mask

Rich in vitamin E—a powerful antioxidant—avocados are great for nourishing the skin and are almost as good taken externally as internally. Take 1 ripe avocado and mash the flesh in a bowl with a fork. When it's a soft paste, apply to the face, avoiding the eyes. Don't throw the stone away! Use it to gently massage the pulp over your skin, moving the stone over your face in slow circles. Leave for five minutes. Wash off your face with warm water and massage in your favorite moisturizer.

45 Deep-tension disperser

This can be performed whenever you need a quick stress reliever. It loosens tension in the scalp and helps counteract any unconscious frowning you might be doing that leads to lines on the face, especially across the forehead and between the bridge of your nose. Close your eyes and with the pads of the fingers of both hands start making small circular movements at your forehead. Move upward to your hairline and as if along a center parting back to the nape of your neck. Work forward along each side of your head to the forehead, then back again. Repeat until the whole head has been massaged. Concentrate on moving the scalp, not the hair.

46 Yoga for youth

Yoga massages your internal organs, helping them function optimally, which supports your other efforts to detox. So if you've been meaning to invest in a book or video and begin your own practice, make today the day. Alternatively, try the two moves that follow. The Plough increases energy and improves the circulation, so it will help skin condition and flexibility. The Fish is a counterstretch to the Plough and should always follow it. If you have a medical condition, neck problems, or are pregnant, give these a miss.

47 The Plough

Lie on your back, arms by your sides, and breathe in as you
bring your knees to your chest. Breathe out and straighten
your legs, taking them upward and using your hands to
support your back and push yourself a little higher. Take your
legs over your head and, if you can, place your feet on the
floor with toes curled under, legs straight, and arms now flat
on the floor by your side. If you can't put your feet on the
floor, continue to use your arms to support your back and try
to maintain balance. Take several deep breaths, then when
ready, gradually unroll your spine, bringing your legs back
up in the air and finally
flat on the floor.

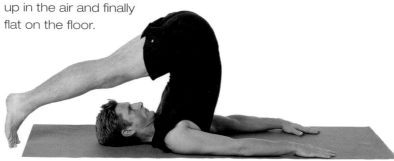

48 The Fish

When you are back in the start position, arch your back, supporting yourself on your elbows with your lower arms flat on the floor, palms facing down. Your head will have lifted off the floor. Now lower gently downward so that the top of your head is on the floor. Hold the position, then slide your neck and head back to the floor. Relax.

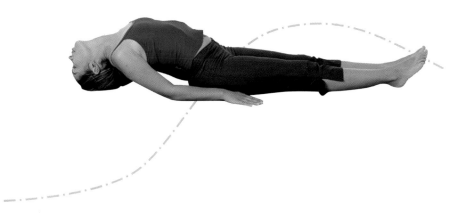

49 Healing olive manicure

Olive oil soothes hands and softens cuticles. Heat 2 tbsp olive oil very gently until slightly warm to the touch but not too hot. Remove old nail varnish, soak and dry hands, rub a little olive oil into your cuticles, and gently ease back with an orange stick tipped with cotton wool or a Q-Tip. Massage a teaspoon of olive oil into your hands. Then find the acupressure point "heart 7." With your palm facing up, draw an imaginary line from your ring finger to your wrist. The point where the line and wrist crease meet is "heart 7." Support your left hand with your right hand and apply pressure on the point with your right thumb. Press for a second, release for a second. Continue for one minute, then repeat on the right hand.

50 Dinner: powerhouse salad (requires pre-preparation)

This amazingly nutritious salad boosts the immune system, raises energy levels, and, because it replaces the vitamin C that stress depletes, helps tissue repair.

Take 1 medium can of chickpeas, drained and rinsed, or the equivalent dry weight, roughly 14oz (400g), soaked and ready to eat. Combine with half a chopped red onion, half 1 red capsicum pepper, and a handful of fresh chopped coriander. Make a dressing with 1 crushed

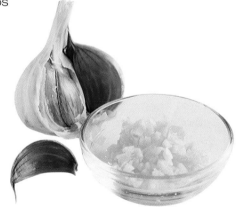

garlic clove, 2 tbsp olive oil, and the juice of 1 lime. Pour over salad. Leave for an hour before eating.

51 Cherishing peppermint pedicure

Activating reflexology points in the soles of your feet rebalances the entire body. Slough off dead skin with a pumice. Add 10 drops tea tree oil (which is antibacterial) to a basin of warm water. Soak your feet for ten minutes, then massage them or roll them on a foot-massage roller. Give each foot at least five minutes' attention. Then massage in some lotion to which you have added a drop or two of soothing and refreshing peppermint oil. Wrap your feet in a towel and lie with feet elevated for 20 minutes. When the lotion is dry, paint your toenails if you like. When the varnish is dry, apply another layer of peppermint lotion, slip on some cotton socks and retire. Tomorrow you'll be walking on air and won't be able to stop staring at your pretty, smooth feet.

Purify

Choose this program when you've been overindulging . . . when you're overloaded and overwhelmed . . . when your physical health has slipped way down your list of priorities.

Today you'll take a rest from solid foods and enjoy pure juices. The theory is the same as with traditional detoxing fasts: by relieving your body of physical stress you free it up to begin to work more efficiently to restore you to health. Mental stress encourages a build-up of toxic by-products that cause ill-health. This program is designed as a retreat for your mind as well as a rest for your body.

By tomorrow you'll feel light and bright and ready to face the world again.

52 Breakfast: carrot and apple juice

Loaded with betacarotene and vitamin C, this is gentle on the system but packs a powerful antioxidant punch. Juice together 4 carrots and 2 apples. Purists will sip it at room temperature (less stressful for your digestive system) but you may prefer to add a couple of chunks of ice.

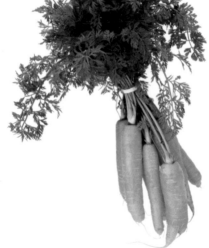

53 Aromatic stone steam

This is based on an ancient Indian remedy used to help those with respiratory disease (and it is excellent any time you are "blocked up" because of a cold, hayfever, or sinusitis). Fill a small bowl with pebbles and little stones. Add 10 drops eucalyptus oil, 10 drops tea tree oil, and 10 drops peppermint or pine oil. Place the bowl in your shower where it won't be in the direct line of the water flow. Set the shower to hot and leave it to run. When the shower is seriously steamy, the fragrance will be released. Now enter the shower. Take deep breaths and feel the scented steam enter right into your lungs, opening up your airways.

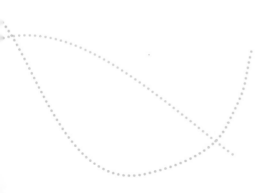

54 Invigorating rosemary scalp massage and lemon rinse

Rosemary essential oil is antiseptic and good for restoring focus and energy. Add 3 drops rosemary oil to 2 tbsp almond or other base oil. If your hair is short, this may be enough for the massage; if long, add the oils to 1 tbsp normal conditioner and blend well. Drench hair, towel dry, and massage the rosemary blend into your scalp. Start from the hair-line—front, sides, and back in turn—and slowly work toward the center of your head each time with the pads of your fingers. Concentrate on the scalp, not the hair. Put on a shower cap or wrap hair in a towel and leave for ten minutes. Rinse well and finish with a lemon rinse of 3½ U.S. pints (2 liters) cool water with the juice of a lemon squeezed into it to close the hair cuticles and give your hair shine.

55 Detoxing exfoliation

Salt is one of the great purifiers. Use Epsom salts (available from chemists), Dead Sea salts, or sea salt flakes. Make sure any scratches are covered with a plaster before beginning. Take a cup of salts and add enough water to make a thick paste. Massage the paste vigorously over your skin, using a flannel or loofah, then rinse off in cool water. Wrap yourself in warm towels or a toweling robe and lie down while you sip a large glass of water.

56 Balancing massage

After exfoliating, this massage will nourish skin. You will need 1¼ tbsp (25 ml) almond oil, 5 drops rosemary essential oil, 5 drops juniper essential oil, and 5 drops geranium essential oil. This combination is purifying and balancing, calming yet invigorating, and it boosts the circulation so is a good detoxifier. Massage the oil into your body from your toes up to your neck (not your face) with long, even strokes. Work into tension points with your thumbs and fingers. Wrap up in a toweling robe.

57 Resting wrap

Pop on some snuggly socks and wrap your head in a towel so that you don't lose body heat. Lay two or three blankets on the bed, lie on them, and wrap them tightly around you (it's even better if someone else can do this for you). Make sure that you have a comfy, plump pillow to rest your head on. Now, cocooned and cozy, doze until lunchtime. (If you have used the oil mix recommended above, you may be too stimulated to nap, in which case, climb into bed and read an uplifting book.)

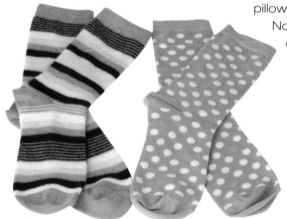

58 Lunch: vegetable zinger

Juicing is a great way of concentrating the nutrients from a serious amount of vegetables into one drink. Much easier than ploughing your way through a plate of food!

This vegetable juice is rich in micronutrients that restore health. Juice 2 broccoli florets, 1 cauliflower floret, 1 celery stick, 1 tomato, 2 carrots, 1 garlic clove, and 1 dtsp olive oil or flaxseed oil.

You can now feel virtuous as you've consumed the recommended daily amount of vegetables in just one glass of juice.

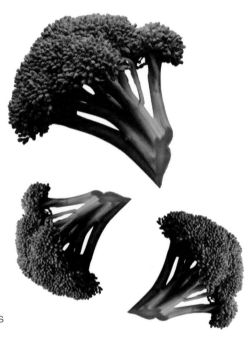

59 Attitude makeover

Do you have the energy and focus that you'd like? Today take some time to explore why you were drawn to the Purify program. Spend an hour this afternoon with your journal. Write a page "free form," exploring your feelings about your health and your attitude to self-care. Do you want to cut down on caffeine, nicotine, or alcohol? Do you know that exercise is vital but never have time to do any? Do you live a stressful life with little or no "me-time?" Formulate plans to incorporate these life-saving strategies into your routine and work out methods of avoiding those situations in which you are tempted to overindulge in bad habits. Read helpful books for ideas. Resolve that today will be the first day of a new and healthier way of living.

60 Glorious mud bath

Therapeutic mud has a particularly high mineral content that helps draw out toxins trapped in the skin. It also has a stimulating effect on the circulation, which helps the detoxing process further. An added bonus is that it's a hoot to use and guaranteed to bring out your "inner child." If the weather is warm, don a bikini, go out into the garden or on your balcony, and slather yourself with a therapeutic mud from a health store or chemist. Have a true "sun bath" and allow the sun's heat and gentle breeze to dry the mud. Shower off with warm water and moisturize with a nourishing body lotion. If the weather is cold, revel in a therapeutic mud bath. (Again, you can buy one in a health store; Moors mud or Dead Sea mud are particularly good.)

61 Dinner: soothing smoothie

This is filling and delicious and full of potassium, essential for dealing with the physical signs of stress. Blend 1 banana, half a honeydew melon (deseeded), 4 fresh apricots (stones removed), and a handful of strawberries. Sip slowly.

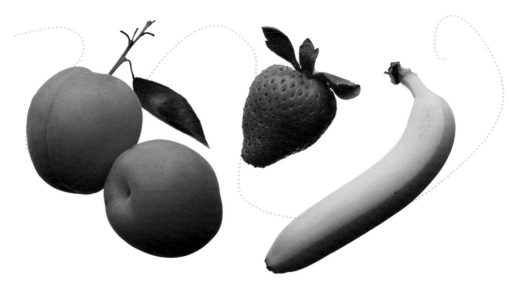

62 White-light protection remedy

When you are left feeling frustrated, harried, or diminished by other people's negativity, this is a marvelous meditation. Its main purpose is to leave you feeling centered and cleansed; its side effect is to throw a protective "aura" around you to make you feel protected and secure. Sit quietly, breathing from your abdomen. Imagine a pinpoint of white light entering through the crown of your head. As it enters imagine it fanning out until a cascade of white light is pouring through your body, purifying and strengthening. Now imagine the white cascade turning slowly into a cloud of protective rose-pink light surrounding your body. See that the pink cloud is emanating from your heart. Stay with this until the image is strong. With practice you will be able to conjure up this protective pink cloud at will and use it to deflect negativity.

63 Instant detox [5]

Detox your teabreak by switching to a caffeine-free tea. Dandelion tea has high levels of potassium, which helps neutralize the effect of salt in the diet and also increases production of detoxifying enzymes in the liver. Green tea has high levels of antioxidants. There is also some research that shows it may cut by up to a third the production of enzymes that encourage the body to store fat, so it is particularly useful for those who are bothered by cellulite.

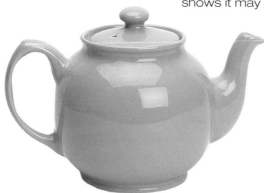

Rescue

Choose this program when you have forgotten what it's like not to feel stressed . . . when looking at your "to do" list fills you with panic . . . when your body is beginning to let you down because stress has drained you of strength and energy.

The program for today will help you unwind and leave you serene. When burnout threatens it's essential to shift the emphasis on to mind-body therapies that work on a deep level to release tension and calm your mind. Stress depletes vitamin C, necessary for a healthy immune system, and that makes you more prone to illness. Today you'll rectify that with a diet of raw foods.

By tomorrow you will feel rested, stronger, and more in control.

64 Deeply calming yogic breathing

Light a candle. Sit comfortably, preferably cross-legged on the floor. Don't slouch—be conscious of your spine supporting your body and keep your shoulders down and relaxed. Your hands should rest on your knees, palms upward. Now bend the three middle fingers of your left hand into the palm, with the thumb and little finger sticking up. Use your right thumb to block your right nostril. Breathe in deeply for a count of eight and out for a count of eight. Do this ten times, then block your left nostril with your left thumb and repeat for the other side. As thoughts come into your mind, breathe them out on the exhale.

65 Stress-relieving yoga stretch

Kneel so that the backs of your thighs and calves form an "L" and your knees are hip-width apart. Lightly hold your forearms behind your back. Breathe in and on the exhale push your hips forward and grasp your heels with your hands. (If you can't manage this, keep holding your forearms.) Relax your head and neck backward to form an arch. Hold for a count of ten, breathing deeply. Slowly sit down on your heels, and follow with the position on the next page. If you struggle with this exercise at first, don't be despondent. Practise on a daily basis and you'll be impressed by how quickly your muscles loosens up. Avoid this and the next position if you are pregnant.

66 Child's pose

Adopt the Child's pose by sitting with your knees bent and legs tucked under you. Bend forward so your forehead rests on the floor in front of you. Your arms should lie by your sides with hands pointing back and palms upward. Breathe deeply and maintain for several minutes if you can. You may find it more comfortable if you place a pillow on your knees. Stay for as long as is comfortable. The Child's pose is good for relieving tension in your neck and shoulders.

67 Breakfast: live shake

Combine and blend 9oz (250g) live natural yogurt, 1 banana, and a handful or two of other soft fruits such as peach, mango, strawberries, or pineapple. Live yogurt has been shown to help in combating stress-related gut problems and the banana is high in potassium, which is necessary to balance blood pressure. The other fruits will supply vitamin C. This shake is thick, so add a few spoonfuls of fruit juice as well if you like.

68 Sky-gazing

It is estimated that 90 percent of Westerners spend 90 percent of their time inside. Yet Japanese academic studies attest to the fact that being in the open air, preferably feeling close to nature, is beneficial for our well-being and mental health. So today, do yoga stretches in your garden, eat lunch al fresco, or go for a walk in your local park. Alternatively, simply lie on the grass somewhere and relax. Spend as much time as possible outside—the whole morning ideally. Take time to really look at the sky, losing yourself in the cloud formations and changes of color as the day progresses.

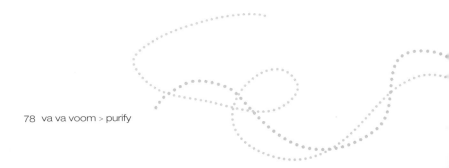

69 Rewrite your internal "script"

Toxic thoughts can be almost as detrimental to your mental health as a toxic environment is to your physical state, but many of us go through life with our mind in a "soup" of toxicity. Jot down some of the thoughts you've had in the past few days relating to your attitude, intelligence, motivation, body, and relationships. You'll see for yourself what we're getting at. Your mind will always respond to the stronger of two thoughts. If you think "I can't cope," that is the reality you will create. Take a few minutes to write down some positive statements—always in the present tense. Try "I am directing my life the way I want it to be," "I am coping beautifully with everything life throws at me," and "Every day I look better because I look after my health." Repeat these to yourself every couple of hours throughout the day—and remind yourself of at least one every day from now on.

70 Lunch: anti-stress salad (requires pre-preparation)

Stress depletes vitamin C; this colorful salad replaces it. Take a half each of 1 red, 1 green, and 1 yellow capsicum pepper, deseed them, split them in half to make quarters, brush with olive oil, and grill (skin side up) until the skins blacken. Leave to cool, then peel off the skins and cut into strips. (Immersing the peppers in cold water speeds up this process, but you need to blot them after with kitchen towel.) Make a marinade with 1 tbsp olive oil, 1 dtsp balsamic vinegar, a squeeze of lemon, and 1 crushed garlic clove. Put some rocket leaves into a bowl, toss in the peppers, and spoon over the marinade. Chill for an hour before serving.

71 Zen ritual

The Japanese bath is as much about refreshing the mind and spirit as getting the body clean. This ritual puts you in the "mindful" state and, combined with the following two treatments (Tips 72 and 73), will give you insight into why the Japanese bath is considered a sacred experience. Light an incense stick or an aromatherapy burner and burn a few drops of geranium, frankincense, or lavender essential oil, all of which restore equilibrium. Sit cross-legged or on a chair or stool in a quiet room with your eyes closed, breathing deeply. Lay your hands on your stomach and feel it rise and fall with each breath. Let go of all other thoughts. Be conscious of the evidence of your senses—what you can hear, smell, feel—and when anxious thoughts come into your mind, let them drift away in the fragrance rising from the burner. This is the "mindful" state. Hold on to it.

72 Serenity scrub

Take the diffuser into the bathroom. Set the shower to a slightly cooler temperature than you would normally have. First body brush (see Tip 1) then step under the water jet. Repeat the movements of dry skin brushing but this time with a loofah or sisal glove and soap to really cleanse and exfoliate your skin. While you are showering, stay in the "mindful" state. When thoughts intrude imagine them becoming plastered to your skin, then being softly peeled away and disappearing with the water. Shampoo your hair. Step out of the shower and wrap yourself up in soft towels, ready for the next part of your ritual.

73 Japanese drench

The purpose of this bath is not to get clean but to meditate. Run a warm bath adding a few drops of your chosen balancing oil (see Tip 71). Step into the bath and sink down in the water. Adopt the mindful state and concentrate on your breathing for a few minutes. Then, using a small bowl, gently and slowly ladle water over your arms, back, and head. Drench your whole body, concentrating fully on the sensations of the water on your skin and the sight of the water running over your body. Continue until a rhythm is developed and you are in a sort of trance. When you have reached this state, soak for a little longer. Let your mind stay clear. Step out of the bath, wrap yourself in warm towels, and, when dry, dress in comforting, comfortable clothes.

74 Restorative tea ritual

Just as the bathing ritual is not just about getting clean, the tea ritual is not just about having a cup of tea. It is a form of meditation designed to still and quiet the mind. Invent your own version. You will need a tea that you enjoy—herbal is fine, but using loose leaf tea (green tea is best) will seem more authentic. Light a candle in a cozy corner of your home and then make your tea, slowly, carefully maintaining the mindful state, concentrating on every action. Now settle down in your corner with your tea and sip it slowly. Use the candle flame as a focus of your attention along with the taste of the tea. Think only of these things and when other thoughts come, visualize them drifting away in the fragrant steam of your tea.

75 Instant detox [6]

Detox grocery shopping. Buy organic when at all possible.
If you can only afford to buy some organic items, current
opinion is that you should prioritize organic dairy products
first, then organic poultry and meat, and then organic
vegetables. Always wash and peel vegetables and fruit,
even if it's not organic. Look for yogurt with the words
"lactobacillus" and "bifidobacterium," which should indicate
those containing live bacteria that fight disease and boost
immunity. Buy organic dried fruits when detoxing to avoid
the chemicals often used to preserve them.

76 Laughter therapy

After the Zen ritual, it's time to change the pace. No more mindful concentration—now for some mindless indulgence. Snuggle down in bed or on the couch with a warm blanket and watch a video of a favorite comedy program or movie for at least an hour. Choose one that you find laugh-out-loud funny. Laughter is a wonderful stress reliever. It releases hormones in the brain that make you feel better and there is research to show that the physical act of laughing massages the inner organs and improves their function.

77 Dinner: elimination salad

Beansprouts are helpful in stimulating the elimination of toxins. They are also incredibly easy to grow if you fancy growing your own. Capsicum peppers help improve circulation and are rich in vitamin C. Take two handfuls of beansprouts, half 1 red pepper, half 1 yellow pepper, a cupful of white cabbage (finely shredded), and the juice of 1 orange. Mix these together and serve. Alternatively, omit the orange juice and flash-fry the ingredients in a little olive oil in a wok.

78 Sleep-inducing facial

This aromatherapy facial relaxes tension in your face and should help you sleep. You will need 3½ tbsp (50ml) almond or other base oil, 10 drops lavender essential oil, and 10 drops ylang ylang essential oil. Lavender is comforting, restorative, and tension-dissolving. Ylang ylang is soothing and balancing. This will make more than you need for this facial, so keep the remainder in a clean, dark glass bottle for future use. Pour a few drops onto your palms, rub them, and cup your hands over your face. Take slow abdominal breaths. Using your forefingers, with small circular movements massage between your eyes, your temples, either side of your nostrils, the dimple of your chin, the corners of your mouth, and then back to the temples.

Restore

Choose this program when you're recovering from illness or trauma, grieving, or feeling otherwise emotionally drained . . . when you're spiritually exhausted . . . when you are mourning the loss of health, love, or a dream.

If this is your state of mind, treating yourself gently is all important—do nothing harsh, demanding, or challenging. This program will restore strength, nurture your sense of self, and promote peace of mind.

By tomorrow you will feel a little comforted, a little stronger, and a lot more rested.

79 Breakfast: cozy oatmeal

Oatmeal is rich in the B vitamins that keep your nervous system healthy and help you combat stress in the long term. Combine a cupful of organic oatmeal with water according to the directions on the packet and stir until ready. Mix with a large dollop of live yogurt (supplying protein for energy), a handful of dried apricots or sultanas, and 1 tsp honey if you like your oatmeal sweet. (Honey is one of the easiest foods for the body to digest.)

80 The loving hands massage

This is based on abhyanga ("loving hands"), an ayurvedic treatment that involves being massaged by two therapists simultaneously. You can recreate the "loving intention" if not the actual treatment at home by massaging yourself not once but twice. You will need 7 tbsp (100ml) sesame oil in a small plastic container. Place the container in a bowl of hot water. When it feels pleasantly warm, using small circular movements, massage the oil into your skin beginning with the soles of your feet, then work upward covering your whole body, always working toward the heart. Work between your toes, behind your ears, round your bellybutton—everywhere. Try to enter a meditative state where you concentrate on nothing but nourishing your body and appreciating its strength and beauty. Then repeat the massage, but more slowly, more thoughtfully.

81 Lunch: comfort food

The hormone dopamine keeps you on an even keel. For this you need vitamin B12, which you can get from chicken. Grill a breast of organic, free-range chicken and serve with mashed potato (softened with a little olive oil) and heaps of green beans and broccoli. If you're vegetarian, grate some cheese over the potato instead of the chicken.

82 Herbal help

Milk thistle is a gentle restorative herb that helps the liver perform its vital detoxifying function. It promotes the work of a compound called glutathione that speeds up the removal of toxins. Take around 150mg three times a day regularly to receive benefits. However, to give your liver a powerful restorative boost today, take 300mg in the morning and again in the evening. Milk thistle is available from health food stores.

83 Restoration exfoliaton

Honey is making a comeback in our hospital wards as medics rediscover its potent antibacterial and healing powers. Combine 4 tsp clear, runny honey, 2 drops lavender essential oil, and 2 drops rose essential oil in a small bowl. Thoroughly cleanse your face and apply this exfoliation mixture to your face, neck, and décolletage. Leave it on for 10 minutes, then gently rub over the areas with your fingers to remove it. Sweep away any residue with cotton wool dipped in tepid water.

84 Complexion resurrection

Combine 5 drops rose essential oil and 5 drops lavender essential oil in 1½ tbsp (25ml) almond or other base oil. Gently massage the mixture into your face, neck, and décolletage. Leave it on while you follow with Tip 86 or for 20 minutes, then remove it with cotton wool soaked in tepid water.

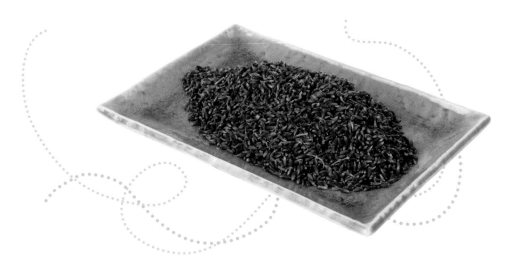

85 Dinner: meditation soup (requires pre-preparation)

Chop and prepare all the ingredients beforehand, placing them in little piles in separate bowls or plates. Concentrate on your actions, the pleasing aspect of the ingredients, and the pleasure to be derived from cooking a simple, nourishing meal for yourself. In a large saucepan gently fry in 1 tbsp olive oil or rapeseed oil, 1 onion, 1 crushed garlic clove, half a tsp grated ginger, and half a leek, until soft. Add 1 U.S. pint (500ml) vegetable stock, a handful of frozen peas, 1 chopped carrot, 1 chopped potato, and a medium can of drained and rinsed lentils (or chickpeas). Bring to the boil and simmer for around 15 minutes until all the ingredients are cooked. Liquidize. Scatter a few leaves of fresh parsley on top, season with black pepper, and serve.

86 Chamomile eye rescue

Chamomile is wonderful for soothing tired, overworked eyes (or eyes red from crying). Use cooled, used chamomile tea bags over your eyes, or, better still, make your own compresses by adding 1 drop of chamomile essential oil to a mug of hot water. Dilute this with cool water until the total volume is 1½ U.S. pints (1 liter). This water should now be cool enough not to burn delicate skin. Soak two large cotton wool pads in the chamomile water to make compresses. Gently press out excess water, but leave them still quite moist. Dab a few dots of your favorite eye cream around the socket along the bone. (Never apply night cream right under the eyes as it will make them puffy.) Then place the compresses (or tea bags) on top. Now relax for at least 15 minutes before removing them.

87 Love bath

This blissful bath is healing when you have argued with a loved one. It helps you think straight after you've taken an emotional battering. To a hot bath add 5 drops rose essential oil (to open your heart and lift depression), 5 drops rosemary essential oil (to stimulate loving thoughts), and 5 drops sandalwood essential oil (to calm the nervous system). Light candles carefully all around the bathroom. Sink into the bath, relax, and imagine a pink rose in the center of your chest slowly opening and bathing you in pink, healing light. Now imagine any disappointment in your life or your relationship being replaced with understanding and positivity.

88 Let go

Depression can be the result of repressed resentment or anger. When you feel that life has dealt you the wrong card, try to get in touch with the anger that often lies buried deep under a stoic front. Write a short story—three or four pages in which the central character has experienced the same emotions as you. Don't think too hard about it—no one else will read it—but you might find out that freeing yourself up to write like this will uncover some interesting perspectives. Read your story carefully, and think about it. Then take it outside with a box of matches and set it on fire (safely in a brazier or metal bin).

89 Instant detox [7]

Detox your mind. Thoughts are toxic if they lead to stress because stress causes your body to be flooded with adrenaline. This in turn triggers the release of substances that cause undesirable body changes—high blood pressure, blood vessel damage, and even fat accumulation. If you're a worrywart, try to take serious steps to lose the habit and find ways to switch off your anxiety.

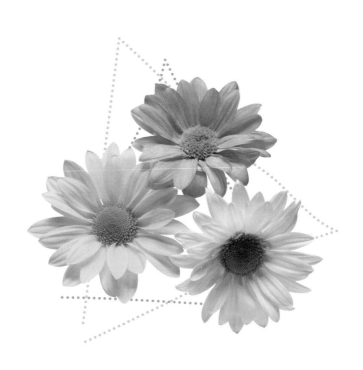

Protect

Choose this program when you're feeling below par . . .
when you succumb to one illness after another . . .
when you are well and want to stay that way.

It relaxes muscles, opens airways, and
boosts your immune system.

To achieve this we use hydrotherapy—the alternate
application of hot and cold water to give a thrilling jolt
to your circulation and hence move your immune
system into a higher gear. You will find it bracing, verging
on the masochistic, but afterward your whole skin will
tingle as if you have just had a dip in the sea. There are
four hydrotherapy treatments in this book; for real
results you need only perform two on any one day. So
read all four and select two.

By tomorrow you will feel reborn!

90 Breakfast: ginger zinger

Ginger is a tonic herb and supports your body's organs. Kiwi fruit is rich in vitamin C to boost your immune system. Cut half a cantaloupe melon into chunks and combine with 1 thinly sliced kiwi fruit and a cupful of grapes (halved). Grate some root ginger until you have half a teaspoon and sprinkle over the fruit. Drizzle over 30ml apple juice. Stir well and enjoy.

91 Scottish douche

We have adapted this treatment so that you can do it at home; at a spa a therapist would treat your spine by directing a jet of water on it with a hose. If possible, adjust your shower to give a narrow, focused jet of water. Turn the temperature to cool and, standing below the showerhead, bend forward and then upright so that the water moves up and down your spine for 90 seconds. This stimulates your parasympathetic nervous system, which originates from your spine and thus affects every organ in your body. Afterward, wrap yourself in warm fluffy towels.

92 Sitz bath

This treatment may seem a little strange and difficult, but it is excellent for the reproductive system. You will need two tubs or basins big enough for you to sit in and old towels or mats to protect the floor from water spillages. Fill one tub with comfortably hot water, the other with cold (the brave add ice cubes). Wear an old T-shirt to keep your top half warm, then lower your bottom into the hot tub. Place your feet in the cold tub. Sit like this for one minute. Now swap— bottom in cold water and feet in hot. Remain like this for one minute. Swap again and repeat twice more until your bottom has been in the hot and cold water three times. Finish by dipping your bottom in hot water and then dry yourself briskly with a towel.

93 Mummy wrap

This is an elaborate treatment but well worth the effort.
You will need an old double sheet cut into strips lengthwise
about 1ft (30cm) wide, a tub or basin, four large towels, and
some plastic sheeting or garbage bags to protect the floor.
Place the tub in the bath or shower tray, fill it with icecubes
and immerse the sheet strips in it. Place the plastic sheeting
on the bathroom floor and lay one of the towels on top.
Now, working quickly, wring out the sheets and wrap them
as tightly as you can around your legs, lower body, torso,
and arms. They should be cold enough to make this feel
unpleasant. Now, wrapping the other towels around you
as tightly as possible (enlist help if necessary), lie down and
relax until the heat of your body has warmed the bandages
and you feel comfortable again (usually around ten minutes).
Unwrap and dry yourself briskly with a towel.

94 Pine inhalation

After the rigors of hydrotherapy, this treatment will warm you. Pine is refreshing and stimulating. Add ten drops pine (or eucalyptus) essential oil to a hot bath. Immerse yourself for at least 20 minutes, breathing deeply. Shut your eyes and imagine you are deep in a pine forest ("seeing" green —the color of healing—is restful in itself). Visualize the pine scent as a refreshing green mist passing deep into your lungs, opening and healing them.

If your mind starts to wander away from the visualization, gently remind yourself to re-focus your thoughts. Concentrate on the mental and physical sensations of warmth and calm that enter you as you visualize the smells and colors. Is the pine smell sharp in your nostrils? How many shades of green can you see in the forest? Taking the time to focus on these kinds of detail help make your visualization experience more intense.

95 Lunch: immunity-boosting salad

Cancer clinics tell their patients to eat almonds every day because of their disease-fighting properties. Iron in beets improves blood function to keep the body free of disease. To make an immunity-boosting salad, you will need 1 or 2 small beets, 1 apple, and a bowl of rocket leaves. Chop up all the ingredients and place them in a bowl. Spread out 1oz (25g) chopped almonds on a baking tray and toast under a grill, turning occasionally, until golden. Toss the almonds in with the vegetables and add a dressing of olive oil and lemon juice.

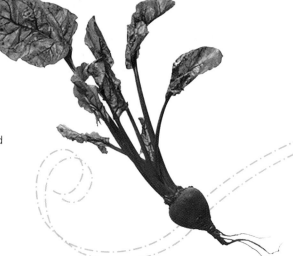

96 Lymph boosting

This afternoon's project is to concentrate on detoxifying your lymphatic system. Just like the circulatory system, the lymph system is a series of tiny vessels passing all through your body, the purpose of which is to carry away the body's waste products so that they can be eliminated. At certain key sites in the lymph glands, white blood cells attack this waste and in this way fight infection. If your lymph system is functioning well, you will rarely succumb to infections. If it's sluggish, you will be vulnerable to frequent illnesses and probably suffer from puffy eyes or ankles. Understanding and caring for your lymph system will improve your health and, since it improves your immune function, potentially add years to your life.

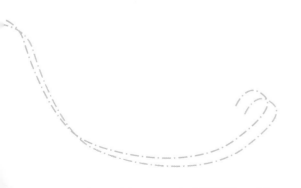

97 Echinacea tonic

Blocked lymph flow can be set moving again with herbs—
echinacea is the prime one. Echinacea boosts the immune
system by increasing the white blood cell count, so it's
invaluable for protecting against disease. Take four drops
(or as directed on the label) echinacea tincture diluted in
water—today and for the next two weeks.

98 Manual lymphatic drainage

Unlike the circulatory system, the lymph system has no heart
to pump lymph around the body. It is moved by the action of
the body's muscles on the vessel walls. A specific form of light
massage—manual lymphatic drainage (MLD)—has been
devised to help the lymphatic system work in prime condition
and if a salon near by offers this, book a session for this
afternoon. Failing that, you can stimulate lymph flow by working
your own muscles. For DIY MLD get outside for a brisk walk,
pumping your arms as you do so. Swimming is also superb.

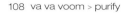

99 Rosemary drench

Rosemary essential oil is excellent for lymph stimulation. Try this naturopathic bath. Add ten drops rosemary essential oil to a warm bath and lie back and relax. After a few minutes, add some cold water and relax again. Repeat, gradually adding cold water until the bath is cool. The change from hot to cold stimulates the lymph, as does the rosemary, making this an extremely effective double treatment.

100 Dinner: reviving risotto

This rice dish is rich in antioxidants, especially betacarotene, which the body converts to vitamin A. Chicken is rich in lysine, which has antiviral properties. If you're vegetarian, simply omit it.

Gently fry a chopped chicken breast in a little oil. In another pan heat 1 tbsp olive oil, then add half an onion, 1 chopped garlic clove, half 1 green capsicum pepper, and half 1 red chilli pepper, (deseeded and chopped). Fry gently until all the ingredients are softening. Add some fresh thyme or a bay leaf and a grind of black pepper and fry for another two minutes or so. Add 3 1/2oz (100g) arborio rice and stir until all the rice is coated. Add 7floz (200ml) vegetable stock, half a medium can tinned tomatoes, and the partially cooked chicken. Cook slowly (for about 20 minutes) until all the fluid has been absorbed by the rice and the chicken is cooked through. You will have to add extra water—do this gradually as needed.

101 Instant detox [8]

A simple way to purify for life? Have one meal a day that is raw and vegetable based.

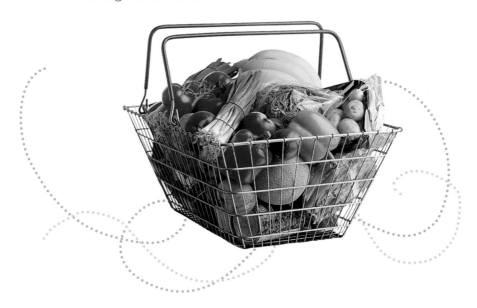

Resources

Books
Detox Solutions, **Helen Foster**
Home Health Sanctuary, **Anna Selby**
The Total Detox Plan, **Sarah Brewer**
The Natural Year, **Jane Alexander**
Mind, Body, Spirit, **Jane Alexander**